THE POWER PROTOCOL

KATYA KARLOVA

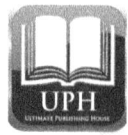

Copyright © 2025 by Ultimate Publishing House

The Power Protocol Journal
Your Weekly Ritual for Reclaiming Power
Author: Katya Karlova

www.KatyaKarlova.com & www.InvisiblePainUnstoppablePower.com

All rights reserved. No part of this journal book may be reproduced in any form or by any means without written permission from the publisher.

Attention: Permissions Coordinator
Ultimate Publishing House
205 Glen Shields Avenue
Toronto, Ontario, Canada
L4K 1T3
Email: info@ultimatepublishinghouse.com

Ultimate Publishing House – Bulk Orders & Corporate Gifting
Looking to elevate your brand or inspire your team? Bulk copies of **The Power Protocol Journal, *Your Weekly Ritual for Reclaiming Power*** are available for companies, organizations, educational institutions, conferences, and client gifting.

Special Incentives for Bulk Orders:

- Orders of 100 copies or more qualify for special pricing.
- Orders of 1,000 copies or more receive deep volume discounts plus a complimentary custom second page featuring your logo, message from the CEO, or brand story — turning this book into a powerful branded asset or client gift.

Whether you're using it for leadership retreats, onboarding, holiday gifts, sponsorship bonuses, or brand awareness campaigns, this book becomes your voice in their hands.

To place a custom bulk order or to discuss tailored publishing solutions:

Call **Ultimate Publishing House:**
📞 1-833-I-LUV-BOOKS (1-833-458-8266) or 647-883-1758
www.ultimatepublishinghouse.com
Email: info@ultimatepublishinghouse.com

The Power Protocol Journal
Your Weekly Ritual for Reclaiming Power
AUTHOR KATYA KARLOVA
Advocate · Speaker · Resilience Coach

ISBN: 979-8-9882088-5-3

THE POWER PROTOCOL

This journal is your companion, your mirror, and your momentum builder. It's designed to help you transform invisible pain into unstoppable power, week by week, reflection by reflection. Remember, this journal is for YOU, there is no judgment here so allow yourself to be completely vulnerable. That is the space that sparks real change.

HOW TO USE THIS JOURNAL

USE WEEKLY SPREADS CONSISTENTLY: Each week offers a repeatable layout- beginning with intention setting and ending with celebration. Fill them in every week for 12 weeks. Feel free to use as you're reading the book or after- often, journaling while reading will allow things to come to the surface we have buried. Good, this journal will help you process them.

HONOR YOUR BODY & EMOTIONS: The "Body Check-In" and "Invisible Pain Tracker" help you tune into what's happening within. Acknowledge but don't judge, there is no right way to heal or grow."

TRANSMUTE, DON'T SUPPRESS: In the "Power Transmutation" section, you'll learn to shift your perspective on pain — and harness it.

CELEBRATE THE SMALL STUFF: The "Wins, Gratitude & Magic Moments" section teaches you to see light — even on the heavy days. Consider creating a mini-ritual for yourself.

LET IT FLOW FREELY: Each week includes a Free Space page. Use it however you need. Healing isn't linear — and neither is creativity.

CLOSE WITH A CEREMONY: The Final section invites you to integrate your growth through letters to your past and future self.

THERE'S NO WRONG WAY TO HEAL: If you miss a day or week — that's okay. This journal doesn't judge.

"LIFE ISN'T ABOUT FINDING YOURSELF.

IT'S ABOUT CREATING YOURSELF."

"Your life does not get better by chance, it gets better by change."

JIM ROHN

MY WEEKLY INTENTION

How am I feeling emotionally, physically & spiritually?
This week, I want to feel… (let this guide your intention)
My core focus:
Support I need this week:

"You are not behind. You are exactly where you're meant to be."

BODY CHECK-IN

What is my body whispering to me?
Physical sensations I've noticed:
Energy highs/lows:
What's calling for attention or rest?

_____

_____

_____

_____

_____

_____

_____

_____

_____

_____

_____

_____

_____

_____

"Success is something you attract by the person you become."

JIM ROHN

INVISIBLE PAIN TRACKER

I'm learning to name what I feel, even when no one sees it.
Pain, tension, or emotional discomfort:
Possible triggers:
My coping responses or support used:

_____

_____

_____

_____

_____

_____

_____

_____

_____

_____

_____

_____

_____

_____

_____

_____

> "Small hinges swing big doors."
> ROBIN SHARMA

POWER TRANSMUTATION

I am transforming pain into power.
What challenge showed up this week?
How can I shift my perspective or response?
A lesson or strength I uncovered:

"What you are not changing, you are choosing."

LAURIE BUCHANAN

WINS, GRATITUDE & MAGIC MOMENTS

1–2 wins this week:
Who or what I'm grateful for:
A magic moment I want to remember:

FREE SPACE / DOODLE / DOWNLOAD PAGE

Use this space however you like — journal, sketch, release, or let something flow through you.

"Discipline is the bridge between goals and accomplishment."
JIM ROHN

MY WEEKLY INTENTION

How am I feeling emotionally, physically & spiritually?
This week, I want to feel… (let this guide your intention)
My core focus:
Support I need this week:

"Your perception creates your reality—choose wisely."

BODY CHECK-IN

What is my body whispering to me?
Physical sensations I've noticed:
Energy highs/lows:
What's calling for attention or rest?

"Your future is created by what you do today, not tomorrow."
ROBERT KIYOSAKI

INVISIBLE PAIN TRACKER

I'm learning to name what I feel, even when no one sees it.
Pain, tension, or emotional discomfort:
Possible triggers:
My coping responses or support used:

"Don't just go through life. Grow through life."
ERIC BUTTERWORTH

POWER TRANSMUTATION

I am transforming pain into power.
What challenge showed up this week?
How can I shift my perspective or response?
A lesson or strength I uncovered:

"Energy flows where attention goes."

BOB PROCTOR

WINS, GRATITUDE & MAGIC MOMENTS

1–2 wins this week:
Who or what I'm grateful for:
A magic moment I want to remember:

FREE SPACE / DOODLE / DOWNLOAD PAGE

Use this space however you like — journal, sketch, release, or let something flow through you.

"You can't outperform your own self-image."

MAXWELL MALTZ

MY WEEKLY INTENTION

How am I feeling emotionally, physically & spiritually?
This week, I want to feel… (let this guide your intention)
My core focus:
Support I need this week:

"In the middle of difficulty lies opportunity."

ALBERT EINSTEIN

BODY CHECK-IN

What is my body whispering to me?
Physical sensations I've noticed:
Energy highs/lows:
What's calling for attention or rest?

"Be so rooted in your purpose that external noise becomes irrelevant."

INVISIBLE PAIN TRACKER

I'm learning to name what I feel, even when no one sees it.
Pain, tension, or emotional discomfort:
Possible triggers:
My coping responses or support used:

"The cave you fear to enter holds the treasure you seek."

JOSEPH CAMPBELL

POWER TRANSMUTATION

I am transforming pain into power.
What challenge showed up this week?
How can I shift my perspective or response?
A lesson or strength I uncovered:

> *"Growth is painful. Change is painful. But nothing is as painful as staying stuck."*
>
> MANDY HALE

WINS, GRATITUDE & MAGIC MOMENTS

1–2 wins this week:
Who or what I'm grateful for:
A magic moment I want to remember:

FREE SPACE / DOODLE / DOWNLOAD PAGE

Use this space however you like — journal, sketch, release, or let something flow through you.

> *"Confidence is not 'they will like me.'*
> *Confidence is 'I'll be fine if they don't.'"*
>
> CHRISTINA GRIMMIE

MY WEEKLY INTENTION

How am I feeling emotionally, physically & spiritually?
This week, I want to feel… (let this guide your intention)
My core focus:
Support I need this week:

....

....

....

....

....

....

....

....

....

....

....

....

....

....

....

"Clarity comes from engagement, not thought."

MARIE FORLEO

BODY CHECK-IN

What is my body whispering to me?
Physical sensations I've noticed:
Energy highs/lows:
What's calling for attention or rest?

> *"Success is not to be pursued; it is to be attracted by the person you become."*
>
> JIM ROHN

INVISIBLE PAIN TRACKER

I'm learning to name what I feel, even when no one sees it.
Pain, tension, or emotional discomfort:
Possible triggers:
My coping responses or support used:

"You are the thinker of your thoughts. Change your thoughts, change your life."

WAYNE DYER

POWER TRANSMUTATION

I am transforming pain into power.
What challenge showed up this week?
How can I shift my perspective or response?
A lesson or strength I uncovered:

"Everything is figureoutable."

MARIE FORLEO

WINS, GRATITUDE & MAGIC MOMENTS

1–2 wins this week:
Who or what I'm grateful for:
A magic moment I want to remember:

FREE SPACE / DOODLE / DOWNLOAD PAGE

Use this space however you like — journal, sketch, release, or let something flow through you.

"When you heal yourself, you heal generations before and after you."

MY WEEKLY INTENTION

How am I feeling emotionally, physically & spiritually?
This week, I want to feel… (let this guide your intention)
My core focus:
Support I need this week:

"Aligned action is the most powerful force in the universe."

ABRAHAM HICKS

BODY CHECK-IN

What is my body whispering to me?
Physical sensations I've noticed:
Energy highs/lows:
What's calling for attention or rest?

_____
_____
_____
_____
_____
_____
_____
_____
_____
_____
_____
_____
_____
_____
_____
_____
_____

"Fall in love with becoming the best version of yourself."

INVISIBLE PAIN TRACKER

I'm learning to name what I feel, even when no one sees it.
Pain, tension, or emotional discomfort:
Possible triggers:
My coping responses or support used:

"Don't be a victim of the world. Be a master of your mind."
JOE DISPENZA

POWER TRANSMUTATION

I am transforming pain into power.
What challenge showed up this week?
How can I shift my perspective or response?
A lesson or strength I uncovered:

"Your vibe attracts your tribe."

WINS, GRATITUDE & MAGIC MOMENTS

1–2 wins this week:
Who or what I'm grateful for:
A magic moment I want to remember:

FREE SPACE / DOODLE / DOWNLOAD PAGE

Use this space however you like — journal, sketch, release, or let something flow through you.

"The mind once stretched by a new idea never returns to its original dimensions."

OLIVER WENDELL HOLMES

MY WEEKLY INTENTION

How am I feeling emotionally, physically & spiritually?
This week, I want to feel… (let this guide your intention)
My core focus:
Support I need this week:

"Act as if it were impossible to fail."

DOROTHEA BRANDE

BODY CHECK-IN

What is my body whispering to me?
Physical sensations I've noticed:
Energy highs/lows:
What's calling for attention or rest?

"Be the energy you want to attract."

INVISIBLE PAIN TRACKER

I'm learning to name what I feel, even when no one sees it.
Pain, tension, or emotional discomfort:
Possible triggers:
My coping responses or support used:

"The most powerful project you'll ever work on is you."

POWER TRANSMUTATION

I am transforming pain into power.
What challenge showed up this week?
How can I shift my perspective or response?
A lesson or strength I uncovered:

"The only way that we can live, is if we grow. The only way that we can grow is if we change."

C. JOYBELL C.

WINS, GRATITUDE & MAGIC MOMENTS

1–2 wins this week:
Who or what I'm grateful for:
A magic moment I want to remember:

FREE SPACE / DOODLE / DOWNLOAD PAGE

Use this space however you like — journal, sketch, release, or let something flow through you.

"Change is the end result of all true learning."

LEO BUSCAGLIA

MY WEEKLY INTENTION

How am I feeling emotionally, physically & spiritually?
This week, I want to feel… (let this guide your intention)
My core focus:
Support I need this week:

> *"If you don't like something, change it. If you can't change it, change your attitude."*
>
> MAYA ANGELOU

BODY CHECK-IN

What is my body whispering to me?
Physical sensations I've noticed:
Energy highs/lows:
What's calling for attention or rest?

"To improve is to change; to be perfect is to change often."
WINSTON CHURCHILL

INVISIBLE PAIN TRACKER

I'm learning to name what I feel, even when no one sees it.
Pain, tension, or emotional discomfort:
Possible triggers:
My coping responses or support used:

> *"If we don't change, we don't grow. If we don't grow, we aren't really living."*
>
> ANATOLE FRANCE

POWER TRANSMUTATION

I am transforming pain into power.
What challenge showed up this week?
How can I shift my perspective or response?
A lesson or strength I uncovered:

> *"Change is the law of life. And those who look only to the past or present are certain to miss the future."*
>
> JOHN F. KENNEDY

WINS, GRATITUDE & MAGIC MOMENTS

1–2 wins this week:
Who or what I'm grateful for:
A magic moment I want to remember:

FREE SPACE / DOODLE / DOWNLOAD PAGE

Use this space however you like — journal, sketch, release, or let something flow through you.

*"We must be willing to let go of the life we planned
so as to have the life that is waiting for us."*

JOSEPH CAMPBELL

MY WEEKLY INTENTION

How am I feeling emotionally, physically & spiritually?
This week, I want to feel... (let this guide your intention)
My core focus:
Support I need this week:

"The only way to make sense out of change is to plunge into it, move with it, and join the dance."

ALAN WATTS

BODY CHECK-IN

What is my body whispering to me?
Physical sensations I've noticed:
Energy highs/lows:
What's calling for attention or rest?

> "When you change the way you look at things, the things you look at change."
>
> WAYNE DYER

INVISIBLE PAIN TRACKER

I'm learning to name what I feel, even when no one sees it.
Pain, tension, or emotional discomfort:
Possible triggers:
My coping responses or support used:

> *"The mind is everything. What you think you become."*
> BUDDHA

POWER TRANSMUTATION

I am transforming pain into power.
What challenge showed up this week?
How can I shift my perspective or response?
A lesson or strength I uncovered:

"The secret of change is to focus all of your energy, not on fighting the old, but on building the new."

SOCRATES

WINS, GRATITUDE & MAGIC MOMENTS

1–2 wins this week:
Who or what I'm grateful for:
A magic moment I want to remember:

FREE SPACE / DOODLE / DOWNLOAD PAGE

Use this space however you like — journal, sketch, release, or let something flow through you.

"Beautiful are those whose brokenness gives birth to transformation and wisdom."

JOHN MARK GREEN

MY WEEKLY INTENTION

How am I feeling emotionally, physically & spiritually?
This week, I want to feel… (let this guide your intention)
My core focus:
Support I need this week:

> *"Change is your friend, not your foe; change is a brilliant opportunity to grow."*
>
> SIMON T. BAILEY

BODY CHECK-IN

What is my body whispering to me?
Physical sensations I've noticed:
Energy highs/lows:
What's calling for attention or rest?

"To transform yourself, you don't need to do big things. Just do small things in a big way. Transformation will follow you."

RAHUL SINHA

INVISIBLE PAIN TRACKER

I'm learning to name what I feel, even when no one sees it.
Pain, tension, or emotional discomfort:
Possible triggers:
My coping responses or support used:

"Transformation literally means going beyond your form."
WAYNE DYER

POWER TRANSMUTATION

I am transforming pain into power.
What challenge showed up this week?
How can I shift my perspective or response?
A lesson or strength I uncovered:

> "Nothing gets transformed in your life
> until your mind is transformed."
>
> IFEANYI ENOCH ONUOHA

WINS, GRATITUDE & MAGIC MOMENTS

1–2 wins this week:
Who or what I'm grateful for:
A magic moment I want to remember:

FREE SPACE / DOODLE / DOWNLOAD PAGE

Use this space however you like — journal, sketch, release, or let something flow through you.

"Change before you have to."

JACK WELCH

MY WEEKLY INTENTION

How am I feeling emotionally, physically & spiritually?
This week, I want to feel… (let this guide your intention)
My core focus:
Support I need this week:

> *"If you resist change, you resist life."*
> SADHGURU

BODY CHECK-IN

What is my body whispering to me?
Physical sensations I've noticed:
Energy highs/lows:
What's calling for attention or rest?

"The only journey is the one within."

RAINER MARIA RILKE

INVISIBLE PAIN TRACKER

I'm learning to name what I feel, even when no one sees it.
Pain, tension, or emotional discomfort:
Possible triggers:
My coping responses or support used:

....

....

....

....

....

....

....

....

....

....

....

....

....

....

....

....

....

"You must be the change you wish to see in the world."
MAHATMA GANDHI

POWER TRANSMUTATION

I am transforming pain into power.
What challenge showed up this week?
How can I shift my perspective or response?
A lesson or strength I uncovered:

> *"When we strive to become better than we are, everything around us becomes better too."*
>
> PAULO COELHO

WINS, GRATITUDE & MAGIC MOMENTS

1–2 wins this week:
Who or what I'm grateful for:
A magic moment I want to remember:

FREE SPACE / DOODLE / DOWNLOAD PAGE

Use this space however you like — journal, sketch, release, or let something flow through you.

"Change is made of choices, and choices are made of character."

AMANDA GORMAN

MY WEEKLY INTENTION

How am I feeling emotionally, physically & spiritually?
This week, I want to feel... (let this guide your intention)
My core focus:
Support I need this week:

"Change brings opportunity."

NIDO QUBEIN

BODY CHECK-IN

What is my body whispering to me?
Physical sensations I've noticed:
Energy highs/lows:
What's calling for attention or rest?

"Sometimes good things fall apart so better things could fall together."

MARILYN MONROE

INVISIBLE PAIN TRACKER

I'm learning to name what I feel, even when no one sees it.
Pain, tension, or emotional discomfort:
Possible triggers:
My coping responses or support used:

....

....

....

....

....

....

....

....

....

....

....

....

....

....

....

....

....

"Only the wisest and stupidest of men never change."
CONFUCIUS

POWER TRANSMUTATION

I am transforming pain into power.
What challenge showed up this week?
How can I shift my perspective or response?
A lesson or strength I uncovered:

"How wonderful it is that nobody need wait a single moment before starting to improve the world."

ANNE FRANK

WINS, GRATITUDE & MAGIC MOMENTS

1–2 wins this week:
Who or what I'm grateful for:
A magic moment I want to remember:

FREE SPACE / DOODLE / DOWNLOAD PAGE

Use this space however you like — journal, sketch, release, or let something flow through you.

"One day or day one. You decide."

UNKNOWN

MY WEEKLY INTENTION

How am I feeling emotionally, physically & spiritually?
This week, I want to feel… (let this guide your intention)
My core focus:
Support I need this week:

"Today was good. Today was fun. Tomorrow is another one."

DR. SEUSS

BODY CHECK-IN

What is my body whispering to me?
Physical sensations I've noticed:
Energy highs/lows:
What's calling for attention or rest?

"Let him that would move the world first move himself."

SOCRATES

INVISIBLE PAIN TRACKER

I'm learning to name what I feel, even when no one sees it.
Pain, tension, or emotional discomfort:
Possible triggers:
My coping responses or support used:

"When we are no longer able to change a situation, we are challenged to change ourselves."

VIKTOR FRANKL

POWER TRANSMUTATION

I am transforming pain into power.
What challenge showed up this week?
How can I shift my perspective or response?
A lesson or strength I uncovered:

"To live is to change. To change is to suffer."

MAXIME LAGACÉ

WINS, GRATITUDE & MAGIC MOMENTS

1–2 wins this week:
Who or what I'm grateful for:
A magic moment I want to remember:

FREE SPACE / DOODLE / DOWNLOAD PAGE

Use this space however you like — journal, sketch, release, or let something flow through you.

> *"Nothing is so painful to the human mind as a great and sudden change."*

MARY WOLLSTONECRAFT SHELLEY

MY WEEKLY INTENTION

How am I feeling emotionally, physically & spiritually?
This week, I want to feel… (let this guide your intention)
My core focus:
Support I need this week:

"All great changes are preceded by chaos."

DEEPAK CHOPRA

BODY CHECK-IN

What is my body whispering to me?
Physical sensations I've noticed:
Energy highs/lows:
What's calling for attention or rest?

"Love change, fear staying the same."

MAXIME LAGACÉ

INVISIBLE PAIN TRACKER

I'm learning to name what I feel, even when no one sees it.
Pain, tension, or emotional discomfort:
Possible triggers:
My coping responses or support used:

"When the winds of change blow, some people build walls and others build windmills."

CHINESE PROVERB

POWER TRANSMUTATION

I am transforming pain into power.
What challenge showed up this week?
How can I shift my perspective or response?
A lesson or strength I uncovered:

> *"Change your thoughts and you change your world."*
> NORMAN VINCENT PEALE

WINS, GRATITUDE & MAGIC MOMENTS

1–2 wins this week:
Who or what I'm grateful for:
A magic moment I want to remember:

FREE SPACE / DOODLE / DOWNLOAD PAGE

Use this space however you like — journal, sketch, release, or let something flow through you.

> *"Nothing happens unless something is moved."*
>
> ALBERT EINSTEIN

MY WEEKLY INTENTION

How am I feeling emotionally, physically & spiritually?
This week, I want to feel… (let this guide your intention)
My core focus:
Support I need this week:

"It's not a setback, it's a setup for growth."

MAXIME LAGACÉ

BODY CHECK-IN

What is my body whispering to me?
Physical sensations I've noticed:
Energy highs/lows:
What's calling for attention or rest?

"If I am an advocate for anything, it is to move. As far as you can, as much as you can. Across the ocean, or simply across the river."

ANTHONY BOURDAIN

INVISIBLE PAIN TRACKER

I'm learning to name what I feel, even when no one sees it.
Pain, tension, or emotional discomfort:
Possible triggers:
My coping responses or support used:

"Only I can change my life. No one can do it for me."
CAROL BURNETT

POWER TRANSMUTATION

I am transforming pain into power.
What challenge showed up this week?
How can I shift my perspective or response?
A lesson or strength I uncovered:

> *"Intelligence is the ability to adapt to change."*
> STEPHEN HAWKING

WINS, GRATITUDE & MAGIC MOMENTS

1–2 wins this week:
Who or what I'm grateful for:
A magic moment I want to remember:

FREE SPACE / DOODLE / DOWNLOAD PAGE

Use this space however you like — journal, sketch, release, or let something flow through you.

"Do not waste time on things you cannot change or influence."

ROBERT GREENE

MY WEEKLY INTENTION

How am I feeling emotionally, physically & spiritually?
This week, I want to feel… (let this guide your intention)
My core focus:
Support I need this week:

"The secret of change is to focus all of your energy, not on fighting the old, but on building the new."

SOCRATES

BODY CHECK-IN

What is my body whispering to me?
Physical sensations I've noticed:
Energy highs/lows:
What's calling for attention or rest?

"Stop being afraid of what could go wrong, and start being excited about what could go right."

TONY ROBBINS

INVISIBLE PAIN TRACKER

I'm learning to name what I feel, even when no one sees it.
Pain, tension, or emotional discomfort:
Possible triggers:
My coping responses or support used:

"The most beautiful and profound way to change yourself is to accept yourself completely, as imperfect as you are."

MAXIME LAGACÉ

POWER TRANSMUTATION

I am transforming pain into power.
What challenge showed up this week?
How can I shift my perspective or response?
A lesson or strength I uncovered:

"The pessimist complains about the wind; the optimist expects it to change; the realist adjusts the sails."

WILLIAM ARTHUR WARD

WINS, GRATITUDE & MAGIC MOMENTS

1–2 wins this week:
Who or what I'm grateful for:
A magic moment I want to remember:

FREE SPACE / DOODLE / DOWNLOAD PAGE

Use this space however you like — journal, sketch, release, or let something flow through you.

"To improve is to change; to be perfect is to change often."
WINSTON CHURCHILL

MY WEEKLY INTENTION

How am I feeling emotionally, physically & spiritually?
This week, I want to feel… (let this guide your intention)
My core focus:
Support I need this week:

"If you want to make enemies, try to change something."
WOODROW WILSON

BODY CHECK-IN

What is my body whispering to me?
Physical sensations I've noticed:
Energy highs/lows:
What's calling for attention or rest?

"Sometimes the winds of change are a hurricane."

DEREK SIVERS

INVISIBLE PAIN TRACKER

I'm learning to name what I feel, even when no one sees it.
Pain, tension, or emotional discomfort:
Possible triggers:
My coping responses or support used:

> *"If you don't like something, change it. If you can't change it, change your attitude."*
>
> MAYA ANGELOU

POWER TRANSMUTATION

I am transforming pain into power.
What challenge showed up this week?
How can I shift my perspective or response?
A lesson or strength I uncovered:

> *"Things do not change; we change."*
> HENRY DAVID THOREAU

WINS, GRATITUDE & MAGIC MOMENTS

1–2 wins this week:
Who or what I'm grateful for:
A magic moment I want to remember:

FREE SPACE / DOODLE / DOWNLOAD PAGE

Use this space however you like — journal, sketch, release, or let something flow through you.

"I alone cannot change the world, but I can cast a stone across the water to create many ripples."

MOTHER TERESA

MY WEEKLY INTENTION

How am I feeling emotionally, physically & spiritually?
This week, I want to feel… (let this guide your intention)
My core focus:
Support I need this week:

"Open your arms to change, but don't let go of your values."
DALAI LAMA

BODY CHECK-IN

What is my body whispering to me?
Physical sensations I've noticed:
Energy highs/lows:
What's calling for attention or rest?

"Your life does not get better by chance, it gets better by change."

JIM ROHN

INVISIBLE PAIN TRACKER

I'm learning to name what I feel, even when no one sees it.
Pain, tension, or emotional discomfort:
Possible triggers:
My coping responses or support used:

"You are not behind. You are exactly where you're meant to be."

POWER TRANSMUTATION

I am transforming pain into power.
What challenge showed up this week?
How can I shift my perspective or response?
A lesson or strength I uncovered:

"Success is something you attract by the person you become."

JIM ROHN

WINS, GRATITUDE & MAGIC MOMENTS

1–2 wins this week:
Who or what I'm grateful for:
A magic moment I want to remember:

FREE SPACE / DOODLE / DOWNLOAD PAGE

Use this space however you like — journal, sketch, release, or let something flow through you.

> *"Small hinges swing big doors."*
>
> ROBIN SHARMA

MY WEEKLY INTENTION

How am I feeling emotionally, physically & spiritually?
This week, I want to feel… (let this guide your intention)
My core focus:
Support I need this week:

"What you are not changing, you are choosing."
LAURIE BUCHANAN

BODY CHECK-IN

What is my body whispering to me?
Physical sensations I've noticed:
Energy highs/lows:
What's calling for attention or rest?

"Discipline is the bridge between goals and accomplishment."
JIM ROHN

INVISIBLE PAIN TRACKER

I'm learning to name what I feel, even when no one sees it.
Pain, tension, or emotional discomfort:
Possible triggers:
My coping responses or support used:

"Your perception creates your reality—choose wisely."

POWER TRANSMUTATION

I am transforming pain into power.
What challenge showed up this week?
How can I shift my perspective or response?
A lesson or strength I uncovered:

"Your future is created by what you do today, not tomorrow."
ROBERT KIYOSAKI

WINS, GRATITUDE & MAGIC MOMENTS

1–2 wins this week:
Who or what I'm grateful for:
A magic moment I want to remember:

FREE SPACE / DOODLE / DOWNLOAD PAGE

Use this space however you like — journal, sketch, release, or let something flow through you.

"Don't just go through life. Grow through life."
ERIC BUTTERWORTH

MY WEEKLY INTENTION

How am I feeling emotionally, physically & spiritually?
This week, I want to feel… (let this guide your intention)
My core focus:
Support I need this week:

"Energy flows where attention goes."

BOB PROCTOR

BODY CHECK-IN

What is my body whispering to me?
Physical sensations I've noticed:
Energy highs/lows:
What's calling for attention or rest?

"You can't outperform your own self-image."

MAXWELL MALTZ

INVISIBLE PAIN TRACKER

I'm learning to name what I feel, even when no one sees it.
Pain, tension, or emotional discomfort:
Possible triggers:
My coping responses or support used:

"In the middle of difficulty lies opportunity."
ALBERT EINSTEIN

POWER TRANSMUTATION

I am transforming pain into power.
What challenge showed up this week?
How can I shift my perspective or response?
A lesson or strength I uncovered:

....

....

....

....

....

....

....

....

....

....

....

....

....

....

"Be so rooted in your purpose that external noise becomes irrelevant."

WINS, GRATITUDE & MAGIC MOMENTS

1–2 wins this week:
Who or what I'm grateful for:
A magic moment I want to remember:

FREE SPACE / DOODLE / DOWNLOAD PAGE

Use this space however you like — journal, sketch, release, or let something flow through you.

"The cave you fear to enter holds the treasure you seek."

JOSEPH CAMPBELL

MY WEEKLY INTENTION

How am I feeling emotionally, physically & spiritually?
This week, I want to feel… (let this guide your intention)
My core focus:
Support I need this week:

> *"Growth is painful. Change is painful. But nothing is as painful as staying stuck."*
>
> MANDY HALE

BODY CHECK-IN

What is my body whispering to me?
Physical sensations I've noticed:
Energy highs/lows:
What's calling for attention or rest?

> *"Confidence is not 'they will like me.'*
> *Confidence is 'I'll be fine if they don't.'"*
>
> CHRISTINA GRIMMIE

INVISIBLE PAIN TRACKER

I'm learning to name what I feel, even when no one sees it.
Pain, tension, or emotional discomfort:
Possible triggers:
My coping responses or support used:

"Clarity comes from engagement, not thought."
MARIE FORLEO

POWER TRANSMUTATION

I am transforming pain into power.
What challenge showed up this week?
How can I shift my perspective or response?
A lesson or strength I uncovered:

> *"Success is not to be pursued; it is to be attracted by the person you become."*
>
> JIM ROHN

WINS, GRATITUDE & MAGIC MOMENTS

1–2 wins this week:
Who or what I'm grateful for:
A magic moment I want to remember:

FREE SPACE / DOODLE / DOWNLOAD PAGE

Use this space however you like — journal, sketch, release, or let something flow through you.

"You are the thinker of your thoughts. Change your thoughts, change your life."

WAYNE DYER

MY WEEKLY INTENTION

How am I feeling emotionally, physically & spiritually?
This week, I want to feel… (let this guide your intention)
My core focus:
Support I need this week:

"Everything is figureoutable."

MARIE FORLEO

BODY CHECK-IN

What is my body whispering to me?
Physical sensations I've noticed:
Energy highs/lows:
What's calling for attention or rest?

"When you heal yourself, you heal generations before and after you."

INVISIBLE PAIN TRACKER

I'm learning to name what I feel, even when no one sees it.
Pain, tension, or emotional discomfort:
Possible triggers:
My coping responses or support used:

"Aligned action is the most powerful force in the universe."
ABRAHAM HICKS

POWER TRANSMUTATION

I am transforming pain into power.
What challenge showed up this week?
How can I shift my perspective or response?
A lesson or strength I uncovered:

"Fall in love with becoming the best version of yourself."

WINS, GRATITUDE & MAGIC MOMENTS

1–2 wins this week:
Who or what I'm grateful for:
A magic moment I want to remember:

FREE SPACE / DOODLE / DOWNLOAD PAGE

Use this space however you like — journal, sketch, release, or let something flow through you.

"Don't be a victim of the world. Be a master of your mind."

JOE DISPENZA

MY WEEKLY INTENTION

How am I feeling emotionally, physically & spiritually?
This week, I want to feel… (let this guide your intention)
My core focus:
Support I need this week:

"Your vibe attracts your tribe."

BODY CHECK-IN

What is my body whispering to me?
Physical sensations I've noticed:
Energy highs/lows:
What's calling for attention or rest?

> *"The mind once stretched by a new idea never returns to its original dimensions."*
>
> OLIVER WENDELL HOLMES

INVISIBLE PAIN TRACKER

I'm learning to name what I feel, even when no one sees it.
Pain, tension, or emotional discomfort:
Possible triggers:
My coping responses or support used:

....

....

....

....

....

....

....

....

....

....

....

....

....

....

....

....

"Act as if it were impossible to fail."

DOROTHEA BRANDE

POWER TRANSMUTATION

I am transforming pain into power.
What challenge showed up this week?
How can I shift my perspective or response?
A lesson or strength I uncovered:

"Be the energy you want to attract."

WINS, GRATITUDE & MAGIC MOMENTS

1–2 wins this week:
Who or what I'm grateful for:
A magic moment I want to remember:

FREE SPACE / DOODLE / DOWNLOAD PAGE

Use this space however you like — journal, sketch, release, or let something flow through you.

"The most powerful project you'll ever work on is you."

MY WEEKLY INTENTION

How am I feeling emotionally, physically & spiritually?
This week, I want to feel… (let this guide your intention)
My core focus:
Support I need this week:

> *"The only way that we can live, is if we grow. The only way that we can grow is if we change."*
>
> C. JOYBELL C.

BODY CHECK-IN

What is my body whispering to me?
Physical sensations I've noticed:
Energy highs/lows:
What's calling for attention or rest?

"Change is the end result of all true learning."
LEO BUSCAGLIA

INVISIBLE PAIN TRACKER

I'm learning to name what I feel, even when no one sees it.
Pain, tension, or emotional discomfort:
Possible triggers:
My coping responses or support used:

> *"If you don't like something, change it. If you can't change it, change your attitude."*
>
> MAYA ANGELOU

POWER TRANSMUTATION

I am transforming pain into power.
What challenge showed up this week?
How can I shift my perspective or response?
A lesson or strength I uncovered:

"To improve is to change; to be perfect is to change often."
WINSTON CHURCHILL

WINS, GRATITUDE & MAGIC MOMENTS

1–2 wins this week:
Who or what I'm grateful for:
A magic moment I want to remember:

FREE SPACE / DOODLE / DOWNLOAD PAGE

Use this space however you like — journal, sketch, release, or let something flow through you.

"If we don't change, we don't grow. If we don't grow, we aren't really living."

ANATOLE FRANCE

MY WEEKLY INTENTION

How am I feeling emotionally, physically & spiritually?
This week, I want to feel... (let this guide your intention)
My core focus:
Support I need this week:

"Change is the law of life. And those who look only to the past or present are certain to miss the future."

JOHN F. KENNEDY

BODY CHECK-IN

What is my body whispering to me?
Physical sensations I've noticed:
Energy highs/lows:
What's calling for attention or rest?

*"We must be willing to let go of the life we planned
so as to have the life that is waiting for us."*

JOSEPH CAMPBELL

INVISIBLE PAIN TRACKER

I'm learning to name what I feel, even when no one sees it.
Pain, tension, or emotional discomfort:
Possible triggers:
My coping responses or support used:

"The only way to make sense out of change is to plunge into it, move with it, and join the dance."

ALAN WATTS

POWER TRANSMUTATION

I am transforming pain into power.
What challenge showed up this week?
How can I shift my perspective or response?
A lesson or strength I uncovered:

> *"When you change the way you look at things, the things you look at change."*
>
> WAYNE DYER

WINS, GRATITUDE & MAGIC MOMENTS

1–2 wins this week:
Who or what I'm grateful for:
A magic moment I want to remember:

FREE SPACE / DOODLE / DOWNLOAD PAGE

Use this space however you like — journal, sketch, release, or let something flow through you.

"The mind is everything. What you think you become."

BUDDHA

MY WEEKLY INTENTION

How am I feeling emotionally, physically & spiritually?
This week, I want to feel… (let this guide your intention)
My core focus:
Support I need this week:

> "The secret of change is to focus all of your energy,
> not on fighting the old, but on building the new."
>
> SOCRATES

BODY CHECK-IN

What is my body whispering to me?
Physical sensations I've noticed:
Energy highs/lows:
What's calling for attention or rest?

> *"Beautiful are those whose brokenness gives birth to transformation and wisdom."*
>
> JOHN MARK GREEN

INVISIBLE PAIN TRACKER

I'm learning to name what I feel, even when no one sees it.
Pain, tension, or emotional discomfort:
Possible triggers:
My coping responses or support used:

*"Change is your friend, not your foe; change
is a brilliant opportunity to grow."*

SIMON T. BAILEY

POWER TRANSMUTATION

*I am transforming pain into power.
What challenge showed up this week?
How can I shift my perspective or response?
A lesson or strength I uncovered:*

"To transform yourself, you don't need to do big things. Just do small things in a big way. Transformation will follow you."

RAHUL SINHA

WINS, GRATITUDE & MAGIC MOMENTS

1–2 wins this week:
Who or what I'm grateful for:
A magic moment I want to remember:

FREE SPACE / DOODLE / DOWNLOAD PAGE

Use this space however you like — journal, sketch, release, or let something flow through you.

"Transformation literally means going beyond your form."

WAYNE DYER

MY WEEKLY INTENTION

How am I feeling emotionally, physically & spiritually?
This week, I want to feel… (let this guide your intention)
My core focus:
Support I need this week:

*"Nothing gets transformed in your life
until your mind is transformed."*

IFEANYI ENOCH ONUOHA

BODY CHECK-IN

What is my body whispering to me?
Physical sensations I've noticed:
Energy highs/lows:
What's calling for attention or rest?

"Change before you have to."

JACK WELCH

INVISIBLE PAIN TRACKER

I'm learning to name what I feel, even when no one sees it.
Pain, tension, or emotional discomfort:
Possible triggers:
My coping responses or support used:

"If you resist change, you resist life."
SADHGURU

POWER TRANSMUTATION

I am transforming pain into power.
What challenge showed up this week?
How can I shift my perspective or response?
A lesson or strength I uncovered:

"The only journey is the one within."

RAINER MARIA RILKE

WINS, GRATITUDE & MAGIC MOMENTS

1–2 wins this week:
Who or what I'm grateful for:
A magic moment I want to remember:

FREE SPACE / DOODLE / DOWNLOAD PAGE

Use this space however you like — journal, sketch, release, or let something flow through you.

"You must be the change you wish to see in the world."

MAHATMA GANDHI

MY WEEKLY INTENTION

How am I feeling emotionally, physically & spiritually?
This week, I want to feel… (let this guide your intention)
My core focus:
Support I need this week:

"When we strive to become better than we are, everything around us becomes better too."

PAULO COELHO

BODY CHECK-IN

What is my body whispering to me?
Physical sensations I've noticed:
Energy highs/lows:
What's calling for attention or rest?

"Change is made of choices, and choices are made of character."
AMANDA GORMAN

INVISIBLE PAIN TRACKER

I'm learning to name what I feel, even when no one sees it.
Pain, tension, or emotional discomfort:
Possible triggers:
My coping responses or support used:

"Change brings opportunity."
NIDO QUBEIN

POWER TRANSMUTATION

I am transforming pain into power.
What challenge showed up this week?
How can I shift my perspective or response?
A lesson or strength I uncovered:

> *"Sometimes good things fall apart so better things could fall together."*
>
> MARILYN MONROE

WINS, GRATITUDE & MAGIC MOMENTS

1–2 wins this week:
Who or what I'm grateful for:
A magic moment I want to remember:

FREE SPACE / DOODLE / DOWNLOAD PAGE

Use this space however you like — journal, sketch, release, or let something flow through you.

"Only the wisest and stupidest of men never change."

CONFUCIUS

MY WEEKLY INTENTION

How am I feeling emotionally, physically & spiritually?
This week, I want to feel… (let this guide your intention)
My core focus:
Support I need this week:

"How wonderful it is that nobody need wait a single moment before starting to improve the world."

ANNE FRANK

BODY CHECK-IN

What is my body whispering to me?
Physical sensations I've noticed:
Energy highs/lows:
What's calling for attention or rest?

"One day or day one. You decide."

UNKNOWN

INVISIBLE PAIN TRACKER

I'm learning to name what I feel, even when no one sees it.
Pain, tension, or emotional discomfort:
Possible triggers:
My coping responses or support used:

"Today was good. Today was fun. Tomorrow is another one."
DR. SEUSS

POWER TRANSMUTATION

I am transforming pain into power.
What challenge showed up this week?
How can I shift my perspective or response?
A lesson or strength I uncovered:

> *"Let him that would move the world first move himself."*
>
> SOCRATES

WINS, GRATITUDE & MAGIC MOMENTS

1–2 wins this week:
Who or what I'm grateful for:
A magic moment I want to remember:

FREE SPACE / DOODLE / DOWNLOAD PAGE

Use this space however you like — journal, sketch, release, or let something flow through you.

"When we are no longer able to change a situation, we are challenged to change ourselves."

VIKTOR FRANKL

MY WEEKLY INTENTION

How am I feeling emotionally, physically & spiritually?
This week, I want to feel… (let this guide your intention)
My core focus:
Support I need this week:

"To live is to change. To change is to suffer."

MAXIME LAGACÉ

BODY CHECK-IN

What is my body whispering to me?
Physical sensations I've noticed:
Energy highs/lows:
What's calling for attention or rest?

"Nothing is so painful to the human mind as a great and sudden change."

MARY WOLLSTONECRAFT SHELLEY

INVISIBLE PAIN TRACKER

I'm learning to name what I feel, even when no one sees it.
Pain, tension, or emotional discomfort:
Possible triggers:
My coping responses or support used:

"All great changes are preceded by chaos."

DEEPAK CHOPRA

POWER TRANSMUTATION

I am transforming pain into power.
What challenge showed up this week?
How can I shift my perspective or response?
A lesson or strength I uncovered:

"Love change, fear staying the same."

MAXIME LAGACÉ

WINS, GRATITUDE & MAGIC MOMENTS

1–2 wins this week:
Who or what I'm grateful for:
A magic moment I want to remember:

FREE SPACE / DOODLE / DOWNLOAD PAGE

Use this space however you like — journal, sketch, release, or let something flow through you.

> "When the winds of change blow, some people build walls and others build windmills."

CHINESE PROVERB

MY WEEKLY INTENTION

How am I feeling emotionally, physically & spiritually?
This week, I want to feel… (let this guide your intention)
My core focus:
Support I need this week:

"Change your thoughts and you change your world."
NORMAN VINCENT PEALE

BODY CHECK-IN

What is my body whispering to me?
Physical sensations I've noticed:
Energy highs/lows:
What's calling for attention or rest?

"Nothing happens unless something is moved."

ALBERT EINSTEIN

INVISIBLE PAIN TRACKER

I'm learning to name what I feel, even when no one sees it.
Pain, tension, or emotional discomfort:
Possible triggers:
My coping responses or support used:

"It's not a setback, it's a setup for growth."

MAXIME LAGACÉ

POWER TRANSMUTATION

I am transforming pain into power.
What challenge showed up this week?
How can I shift my perspective or response?
A lesson or strength I uncovered:

"If I am an advocate for anything, it is to move. As far as you can, as much as you can. Across the ocean, or simply across the river."

ANTHONY BOURDAIN

WINS, GRATITUDE & MAGIC MOMENTS

1–2 wins this week:
Who or what I'm grateful for:
A magic moment I want to remember:

FREE SPACE / DOODLE / DOWNLOAD PAGE

Use this space however you like — journal, sketch, release, or let something flow through you.

"Only I can change my life. No one can do it for me."

CAROL BURNETT

MY WEEKLY INTENTION

How am I feeling emotionally, physically & spiritually?
This week, I want to feel… (let this guide your intention)
My core focus:
Support I need this week:

"Intelligence is the ability to adapt to change."
STEPHEN HAWKING

BODY CHECK-IN

What is my body whispering to me?
Physical sensations I've noticed:
Energy highs/lows:
What's calling for attention or rest?

"Do not waste time on things you cannot change or influence."

ROBERT GREENE

INVISIBLE PAIN TRACKER

I'm learning to name what I feel, even when no one sees it.
Pain, tension, or emotional discomfort:
Possible triggers:
My coping responses or support used:

> *"The secret of change is to focus all of your energy, not on fighting the old, but on building the new."*
>
> SOCRATES

POWER TRANSMUTATION

I am transforming pain into power.
What challenge showed up this week?
How can I shift my perspective or response?
A lesson or strength I uncovered:

"Stop being afraid of what could go wrong, and start being excited about what could go right."

TONY ROBBINS

WINS, GRATITUDE & MAGIC MOMENTS

1–2 wins this week:
Who or what I'm grateful for:
A magic moment I want to remember:

FREE SPACE / DOODLE / DOWNLOAD PAGE

Use this space however you like — journal, sketch, release, or let something flow through you.

"The most beautiful and profound way to change yourself is to accept yourself completely, as imperfect as you are."

MAXIME LAGACÉ

MY WEEKLY INTENTION

How am I feeling emotionally, physically & spiritually?
This week, I want to feel... (let this guide your intention)
My core focus:
Support I need this week:

"The pessimist complains about the wind; the optimist expects it to change; the realist adjusts the sails."

WILLIAM ARTHUR WARD

BODY CHECK-IN

What is my body whispering to me?
Physical sensations I've noticed:
Energy highs/lows:
What's calling for attention or rest?

"To improve is to change; to be perfect is to change often."
WINSTON CHURCHILL

INVISIBLE PAIN TRACKER

I'm learning to name what I feel, even when no one sees it.
Pain, tension, or emotional discomfort:
Possible triggers:
My coping responses or support used:

....

....

....

....

....

....

....

....

....

....

....

....

....

....

....

"If you want to make enemies, try to change something."
WOODROW WILSON

POWER TRANSMUTATION

I am transforming pain into power.
What challenge showed up this week?
How can I shift my perspective or response?
A lesson or strength I uncovered:

"Sometimes the winds of change are a hurricane."

DEREK SIVERS

WINS, GRATITUDE & MAGIC MOMENTS

1–2 wins this week:
Who or what I'm grateful for:
A magic moment I want to remember:

FREE SPACE / DOODLE / DOWNLOAD PAGE

Use this space however you like — journal, sketch, release, or let something flow through you.

"If you don't like something, change it. If you can't change it, change your attitude."

MAYA ANGELOU

MY WEEKLY INTENTION

How am I feeling emotionally, physically & spiritually?
This week, I want to feel… (let this guide your intention)
My core focus:
Support I need this week:

"Things do not change; we change."
HENRY DAVID THOREAU

BODY CHECK-IN

What is my body whispering to me?
Physical sensations I've noticed:
Energy highs/lows:
What's calling for attention or rest?

"I alone cannot change the world, but I can cast a stone across the water to create many ripples."

MOTHER TERESA

INVISIBLE PAIN TRACKER

I'm learning to name what I feel, even when no one sees it.
Pain, tension, or emotional discomfort:
Possible triggers:
My coping responses or support used:

> "Open your arms to change, but don't let go of your values."
> DALAI LAMA

POWER TRANSMUTATION

I am transforming pain into power.
What challenge showed up this week?
How can I shift my perspective or response?
A lesson or strength I uncovered:

"Your life does not get better by chance, it gets better by change."

JIM ROHN

WINS, GRATITUDE & MAGIC MOMENTS

1–2 wins this week:
Who or what I'm grateful for:
A magic moment I want to remember:

FREE SPACE / DOODLE / DOWNLOAD PAGE

Use this space however you like — journal, sketch, release, or let something flow through you.

"You are not behind. You are exactly where you're meant to be."

MY WEEKLY INTENTION

How am I feeling emotionally, physically & spiritually?
This week, I want to feel… (let this guide your intention)
My core focus:
Support I need this week:

"Success is something you attract by the person you become."
JIM ROHN

BODY CHECK-IN

What is my body whispering to me?
Physical sensations I've noticed:
Energy highs/lows:
What's calling for attention or rest?

> *"Small hinges swing big doors."*
> ROBIN SHARMA

INVISIBLE PAIN TRACKER

I'm learning to name what I feel, even when no one sees it.
Pain, tension, or emotional discomfort:
Possible triggers:
My coping responses or support used:

"What you are not changing, you are choosing."
LAURIE BUCHANAN

POWER TRANSMUTATION

I am transforming pain into power.
What challenge showed up this week?
How can I shift my perspective or response?
A lesson or strength I uncovered:

"Discipline is the bridge between goals and accomplishment."
JIM ROHN

WINS, GRATITUDE & MAGIC MOMENTS

1–2 wins this week:
Who or what I'm grateful for:
A magic moment I want to remember:

FREE SPACE / DOODLE / DOWNLOAD PAGE

Use this space however you like — journal, sketch, release, or let something flow through you.

"Your perception creates your reality—choose wisely."

MY WEEKLY INTENTION

How am I feeling emotionally, physically & spiritually?
This week, I want to feel… (let this guide your intention)
My core focus:
Support I need this week:

"Your future is created by what you do today, not tomorrow."
ROBERT KIYOSAKI

BODY CHECK-IN

What is my body whispering to me?
Physical sensations I've noticed:
Energy highs/lows:
What's calling for attention or rest?

"Don't just go through life. Grow through life."
ERIC BUTTERWORTH

INVISIBLE PAIN TRACKER

I'm learning to name what I feel, even when no one sees it.
Pain, tension, or emotional discomfort:
Possible triggers:
My coping responses or support used:

"Energy flows where attention goes."

BOB PROCTOR

POWER TRANSMUTATION

I am transforming pain into power.
What challenge showed up this week?
How can I shift my perspective or response?
A lesson or strength I uncovered:

> *"You can't outperform your own self-image."*
> MAXWELL MALTZ

WINS, GRATITUDE & MAGIC MOMENTS

1–2 wins this week:
Who or what I'm grateful for:
A magic moment I want to remember:

FREE SPACE / DOODLE / DOWNLOAD PAGE

Use this space however you like — journal, sketch, release, or let something flow through you.

"In the middle of difficulty lies opportunity."

ALBERT EINSTEIN

MY WEEKLY INTENTION

How am I feeling emotionally, physically & spiritually?
This week, I want to feel… (let this guide your intention)
My core focus:
Support I need this week:

"Be so rooted in your purpose that external noise becomes irrelevant."

BODY CHECK-IN

What is my body whispering to me?
Physical sensations I've noticed:
Energy highs/lows:
What's calling for attention or rest?

"The cave you fear to enter holds the treasure you seek."
JOSEPH CAMPBELL

INVISIBLE PAIN TRACKER

I'm learning to name what I feel, even when no one sees it.
Pain, tension, or emotional discomfort:
Possible triggers:
My coping responses or support used:

"Growth is painful. Change is painful. But nothing is as painful as staying stuck."

MANDY HALE

POWER TRANSMUTATION

I am transforming pain into power.
What challenge showed up this week?
How can I shift my perspective or response?
A lesson or strength I uncovered:

*"Confidence is not 'they will like me.'
Confidence is 'I'll be fine if they don't.'"*

CHRISTINA GRIMMIE

WINS, GRATITUDE & MAGIC MOMENTS

1–2 wins this week:
Who or what I'm grateful for:
A magic moment I want to remember:

FREE SPACE / DOODLE / DOWNLOAD PAGE

Use this space however you like — journal, sketch, release, or let something flow through you.

"Clarity comes from engagement, not thought."

MARIE FORLEO

MY WEEKLY INTENTION

How am I feeling emotionally, physically & spiritually?
This week, I want to feel… (let this guide your intention)
My core focus:
Support I need this week:

> *"Success is not to be pursued; it is to be attracted by the person you become."*
>
> JIM ROHN

BODY CHECK-IN

What is my body whispering to me?
Physical sensations I've noticed:
Energy highs/lows:
What's calling for attention or rest?

"You are the thinker of your thoughts. Change your thoughts, change your life."

WAYNE DYER

INVISIBLE PAIN TRACKER

I'm learning to name what I feel, even when no one sees it.
Pain, tension, or emotional discomfort:
Possible triggers:
My coping responses or support used:

> *"Everything is figureoutable."*
> MARIE FORLEO

POWER TRANSMUTATION

I am transforming pain into power.
What challenge showed up this week?
How can I shift my perspective or response?
A lesson or strength I uncovered:

_____

_____

_____

_____

_____

_____

_____

_____

_____

_____

_____

_____

_____

_____

_____

_____

"When you heal yourself, you heal generations before and after you."

WINS, GRATITUDE & MAGIC MOMENTS

1–2 wins this week:
Who or what I'm grateful for:
A magic moment I want to remember:

FREE SPACE / DOODLE / DOWNLOAD PAGE

Use this space however you like — journal, sketch, release, or let something flow through you.

"Aligned action is the most powerful force in the universe."
ABRAHAM HICKS

MY WEEKLY INTENTION

How am I feeling emotionally, physically & spiritually?
This week, I want to feel… (let this guide your intention)
My core focus:
Support I need this week:

"Fall in love with becoming the best version of yourself."

BODY CHECK-IN

What is my body whispering to me?
Physical sensations I've noticed:
Energy highs/lows:
What's calling for attention or rest?

"Don't be a victim of the world. Be a master of your mind."

JOE DISPENZA

INVISIBLE PAIN TRACKER

I'm learning to name what I feel, even when no one sees it.
Pain, tension, or emotional discomfort:
Possible triggers:
My coping responses or support used:

....

....

....

....

....

....

....

....

....

....

....

....

....

....

....

....

"Your vibe attracts your tribe."

POWER TRANSMUTATION

*I am transforming pain into power.
What challenge showed up this week?
How can I shift my perspective or response?
A lesson or strength I uncovered:*

_____

_____

_____

_____

_____

_____

_____

_____

_____

_____

_____

_____

_____

_____

_____

> *"The mind once stretched by a new idea never returns to its original dimensions."*
>
> OLIVER WENDELL HOLMES

WINS, GRATITUDE & MAGIC MOMENTS

1–2 wins this week:
Who or what I'm grateful for:
A magic moment I want to remember:

FREE SPACE / DOODLE / DOWNLOAD PAGE

Use this space however you like — journal, sketch, release, or let something flow through you.

"Act as if it were impossible to fail."

DOROTHEA BRANDE

MY WEEKLY INTENTION

How am I feeling emotionally, physically & spiritually?
This week, I want to feel... (let this guide your intention)
My core focus:
Support I need this week:

"Be the energy you want to attract."

BODY CHECK-IN

What is my body whispering to me?
Physical sensations I've noticed:
Energy highs/lows:
What's calling for attention or rest?

"The most powerful project you'll ever work on is you."

INVISIBLE PAIN TRACKER

I'm learning to name what I feel, even when no one sees it.
Pain, tension, or emotional discomfort:
Possible triggers:
My coping responses or support used:

> *"The only way that we can live, is if we grow. The only way that we can grow is if we change."*
>
> C. JOYBELL C.

POWER TRANSMUTATION

I am transforming pain into power.
What challenge showed up this week?
How can I shift my perspective or response?
A lesson or strength I uncovered:

_____
_____
_____
_____
_____
_____
_____
_____
_____
_____
_____
_____
_____
_____
_____

"Change is the end result of all true learning."

LEO BUSCAGLIA

WINS, GRATITUDE & MAGIC MOMENTS

1–2 wins this week:
Who or what I'm grateful for:
A magic moment I want to remember:

FREE SPACE / DOODLE / DOWNLOAD PAGE

Use this space however you like — journal, sketch, release, or let something flow through you.

> *"If you don't like something, change it. If you can't change it, change your attitude."*
>
> MAYA ANGELOU

MY WEEKLY INTENTION

How am I feeling emotionally, physically & spiritually?
This week, I want to feel… (let this guide your intention)
My core focus:
Support I need this week:

"To improve is to change; to be perfect is to change often."

WINSTON CHURCHILL

BODY CHECK-IN

What is my body whispering to me?
Physical sensations I've noticed:
Energy highs/lows:
What's calling for attention or rest?

> *"If we don't change, we don't grow. If we don't grow, we aren't really living."*
>
> ANATOLE FRANCE

INVISIBLE PAIN TRACKER

I'm learning to name what I feel, even when no one sees it.
Pain, tension, or emotional discomfort:
Possible triggers:
My coping responses or support used:

_____
_____
_____
_____
_____
_____
_____
_____
_____
_____
_____
_____
_____
_____
_____
_____

> "Change is the law of life. And those who look only to the past or present are certain to miss the future."
>
> JOHN F. KENNEDY

POWER TRANSMUTATION

I am transforming pain into power.
What challenge showed up this week?
How can I shift my perspective or response?
A lesson or strength I uncovered:

"We must be willing to let go of the life we planned so as to have the life that is waiting for us."

JOSEPH CAMPBELL

WINS, GRATITUDE & MAGIC MOMENTS

1–2 wins this week:
Who or what I'm grateful for:
A magic moment I want to remember:

FREE SPACE / DOODLE / DOWNLOAD PAGE

Use this space however you like — journal, sketch, release, or let something flow through you.

"The only way to make sense out of change is to plunge into it, move with it, and join the dance."

ALAN WATTS

MY WEEKLY INTENTION

How am I feeling emotionally, physically & spiritually?
This week, I want to feel… (let this guide your intention)
My core focus:
Support I need this week:

"When you change the way you look at things, the things you look at change."

WAYNE DYER

BODY CHECK-IN

What is my body whispering to me?
Physical sensations I've noticed:
Energy highs/lows:
What's calling for attention or rest?

> "The mind is everything. What you think you become."
> BUDDHA

INVISIBLE PAIN TRACKER

I'm learning to name what I feel, even when no one sees it.
Pain, tension, or emotional discomfort:
Possible triggers:
My coping responses or support used:

> "The secret of change is to focus all of your energy, not on fighting the old, but on building the new."
>
> SOCRATES

POWER TRANSMUTATION

I am transforming pain into power.
What challenge showed up this week?
How can I shift my perspective or response?
A lesson or strength I uncovered:

> *"Beautiful are those whose brokenness gives birth to transformation and wisdom."*
>
> JOHN MARK GREEN

WINS, GRATITUDE & MAGIC MOMENTS

1–2 wins this week:
Who or what I'm grateful for:
A magic moment I want to remember:

FREE SPACE / DOODLE / DOWNLOAD PAGE

Use this space however you like — journal, sketch, release, or let something flow through you.

"Change is your friend, not your foe; change is a brilliant opportunity to grow."

SIMON T. BAILEY

MY WEEKLY INTENTION

How am I feeling emotionally, physically & spiritually?
This week, I want to feel… (let this guide your intention)
My core focus:
Support I need this week:

"To transform yourself, you don't need to do big things. Just do small things in a big way. Transformation will follow you."

RAHUL SINHA

BODY CHECK-IN

What is my body whispering to me?
Physical sensations I've noticed:
Energy highs/lows:
What's calling for attention or rest?

"Transformation literally means going beyond your form."
WAYNE DYER

INVISIBLE PAIN TRACKER

I'm learning to name what I feel, even when no one sees it.
Pain, tension, or emotional discomfort:
Possible triggers:
My coping responses or support used:

....
....
....
....
....
....
....
....
....
....
....
....
....
....
....
....

*"Nothing gets transformed in your life
until your mind is transformed."*

IFEANYI ENOCH ONUOHA

POWER TRANSMUTATION

*I am transforming pain into power.
What challenge showed up this week?
How can I shift my perspective or response?
A lesson or strength I uncovered:*

"Change before you have to."

JACK WELCH

WINS, GRATITUDE & MAGIC MOMENTS

1–2 wins this week:
Who or what I'm grateful for:
A magic moment I want to remember:

FREE SPACE / DOODLE / DOWNLOAD PAGE

Use this space however you like — journal, sketch, release, or let something flow through you.

"If you resist change, you resist life."

SADHGURU

MY WEEKLY INTENTION

How am I feeling emotionally, physically & spiritually?
This week, I want to feel… (let this guide your intention)
My core focus:
Support I need this week:

_____
_____
_____
_____
_____
_____
_____
_____
_____
_____
_____
_____
_____
_____
_____

"The only journey is the one within."

RAINER MARIA RILKE

BODY CHECK-IN

What is my body whispering to me?
Physical sensations I've noticed:
Energy highs/lows:
What's calling for attention or rest?

"You must be the change you wish to see in the world."

MAHATMA GANDHI

INVISIBLE PAIN TRACKER

I'm learning to name what I feel, even when no one sees it.
Pain, tension, or emotional discomfort:
Possible triggers:
My coping responses or support used:

> *"When we strive to become better than we are, everything around us becomes better too."*
>
> PAULO COELHO

POWER TRANSMUTATION

I am transforming pain into power.
What challenge showed up this week?
How can I shift my perspective or response?
A lesson or strength I uncovered:

....

....

....

....

....

....

....

....

....

....

....

....

....

....

....

"Change is made of choices, and choices are made of character."

AMANDA GORMAN

WINS, GRATITUDE & MAGIC MOMENTS

1–2 wins this week:
Who or what I'm grateful for:
A magic moment I want to remember:

FREE SPACE / DOODLE / DOWNLOAD PAGE

Use this space however you like — journal, sketch, release, or let something flow through you.

"Change brings opportunity."

NIDO QUBEIN

MY WEEKLY INTENTION

How am I feeling emotionally, physically & spiritually?
This week, I want to feel… (let this guide your intention)
My core focus:
Support I need this week:

> *"Sometimes good things fall apart so better things could fall together."*
>
> MARILYN MONROE

BODY CHECK-IN

What is my body whispering to me?
Physical sensations I've noticed:
Energy highs/lows:
What's calling for attention or rest?

"Only the wisest and stupidest of men never change."

CONFUCIUS

INVISIBLE PAIN TRACKER

I'm learning to name what I feel, even when no one sees it.
Pain, tension, or emotional discomfort:
Possible triggers:
My coping responses or support used:

> "How wonderful it is that nobody need wait a single moment before starting to improve the world."
>
> ANNE FRANK

POWER TRANSMUTATION

I am transforming pain into power.
What challenge showed up this week?
How can I shift my perspective or response?
A lesson or strength I uncovered:

> *"One day or day one. You decide."*
>
> UNKNOWN

WINS, GRATITUDE & MAGIC MOMENTS

1–2 wins this week:
Who or what I'm grateful for:
A magic moment I want to remember:

FREE SPACE / DOODLE / DOWNLOAD PAGE

Use this space however you like — journal, sketch, release, or let something flow through you.

"Today was good. Today was fun. Tomorrow is another one."

DR. SEUSS

MY WEEKLY INTENTION

How am I feeling emotionally, physically & spiritually?
This week, I want to feel... (let this guide your intention)
My core focus:
Support I need this week:

"Let him that would move the world first move himself."

SOCRATES

BODY CHECK-IN

What is my body whispering to me?
Physical sensations I've noticed:
Energy highs/lows:
What's calling for attention or rest?

"When we are no longer able to change a situation, we are challenged to change ourselves."

VIKTOR FRANKL

INVISIBLE PAIN TRACKER

I'm learning to name what I feel, even when no one sees it.
Pain, tension, or emotional discomfort:
Possible triggers:
My coping responses or support used:

"To live is to change. To change is to suffer."
MAXIME LAGACÉ

POWER TRANSMUTATION

I am transforming pain into power.
What challenge showed up this week?
How can I shift my perspective or response?
A lesson or strength I uncovered:

> *"Nothing is so painful to the human mind as a great and sudden change."*
>
> MARY WOLLSTONECRAFT SHELLEY

WINS, GRATITUDE & MAGIC MOMENTS

1–2 wins this week:
Who or what I'm grateful for:
A magic moment I want to remember:

FREE SPACE / DOODLE / DOWNLOAD PAGE

Use this space however you like — journal, sketch, release, or let something flow through you.

"All great changes are preceded by chaos."

DEEPAK CHOPRA

MY WEEKLY INTENTION

How am I feeling emotionally, physically & spiritually?
This week, I want to feel… (let this guide your intention)
My core focus:
Support I need this week:

"Love change, fear staying the same."

MAXIME LAGACÉ

BODY CHECK-IN

What is my body whispering to me?
Physical sensations I've noticed:
Energy highs/lows:
What's calling for attention or rest?

> *"When the winds of change blow, some people build walls and others build windmills."*
>
> CHINESE PROVERB

INVISIBLE PAIN TRACKER

I'm learning to name what I feel, even when no one sees it.
Pain, tension, or emotional discomfort:
Possible triggers:
My coping responses or support used:

"Change your thoughts and you change your world."
NORMAN VINCENT PEALE

POWER TRANSMUTATION

I am transforming pain into power.
What challenge showed up this week?
How can I shift my perspective or response?
A lesson or strength I uncovered:

"Nothing happens unless something is moved."

ALBERT EINSTEIN

WINS, GRATITUDE & MAGIC MOMENTS

1–2 wins this week:
Who or what I'm grateful for:
A magic moment I want to remember:

FREE SPACE / DOODLE / DOWNLOAD PAGE

Use this space however you like — journal, sketch, release, or let something flow through you.

"It's not a setback, it's a setup for growth."

MAXIME LAGACÉ

MY WEEKLY INTENTION

How am I feeling emotionally, physically & spiritually?
This week, I want to feel… (let this guide your intention)
My core focus:
Support I need this week:

"If I am an advocate for anything, it is to move. As far as you can, as much as you can. Across the ocean, or simply across the river."

ANTHONY BOURDAIN

BODY CHECK-IN

What is my body whispering to me?
Physical sensations I've noticed:
Energy highs/lows:
What's calling for attention or rest?

_____

_____

_____

_____

_____

_____

_____

_____

_____

_____

_____

_____

_____

_____

_____

_____

_____

"Only I can change my life. No one can do it for me."

CAROL BURNETT

INVISIBLE PAIN TRACKER

I'm learning to name what I feel, even when no one sees it.
Pain, tension, or emotional discomfort:
Possible triggers:
My coping responses or support used:

"Intelligence is the ability to adapt to change."
STEPHEN HAWKING

POWER TRANSMUTATION

I am transforming pain into power.
What challenge showed up this week?
How can I shift my perspective or response?
A lesson or strength I uncovered:

....
....
....
....
....
....
....
....
....
....
....
....
....
....

> *"Do not waste time on things you cannot change or influence."*
> ROBERT GREENE

WINS, GRATITUDE & MAGIC MOMENTS

1–2 wins this week:
Who or what I'm grateful for:
A magic moment I want to remember:

FREE SPACE / DOODLE / DOWNLOAD PAGE

Use this space however you like — journal, sketch, release, or let something flow through you.

"The secret of change is to focus all of your energy, not on fighting the old, but on building the new."

SOCRATES

MY WEEKLY INTENTION

How am I feeling emotionally, physically & spiritually?
This week, I want to feel… (let this guide your intention)
My core focus:
Support I need this week:

"Stop being afraid of what could go wrong, and start being excited about what could go right."

TONY ROBBINS

BODY CHECK-IN

What is my body whispering to me?
Physical sensations I've noticed:
Energy highs/lows:
What's calling for attention or rest?

> "The most beautiful and profound way to change yourself is to accept yourself completely, as imperfect as you are."
>
> MAXIME LAGACÉ

INVISIBLE PAIN TRACKER

I'm learning to name what I feel, even when no one sees it.
Pain, tension, or emotional discomfort:
Possible triggers:
My coping responses or support used:

"The pessimist complains about the wind; the optimist expects it to change; the realist adjusts the sails."

WILLIAM ARTHUR WARD

POWER TRANSMUTATION

I am transforming pain into power.
What challenge showed up this week?
How can I shift my perspective or response?
A lesson or strength I uncovered:

"To improve is to change; to be perfect is to change often."
WINSTON CHURCHILL

WINS, GRATITUDE & MAGIC MOMENTS

1–2 wins this week:
Who or what I'm grateful for:
A magic moment I want to remember:

FREE SPACE / DOODLE / DOWNLOAD PAGE

Use this space however you like — journal, sketch, release, or let something flow through you.

"If you want to make enemies, try to change something."

WOODROW WILSON

MY WEEKLY INTENTION

How am I feeling emotionally, physically & spiritually?
This week, I want to feel… (let this guide your intention)
My core focus:
Support I need this week:

"Sometimes the winds of change are a hurricane."

DEREK SIVERS

BODY CHECK-IN

What is my body whispering to me?
Physical sensations I've noticed:
Energy highs/lows:
What's calling for attention or rest?

_____
_____
_____
_____
_____
_____
_____
_____
_____
_____
_____
_____
_____
_____
_____
_____

> *"If you don't like something, change it. If you can't change it, change your attitude."*
>
> MAYA ANGELOU

INVISIBLE PAIN TRACKER

I'm learning to name what I feel, even when no one sees it.
Pain, tension, or emotional discomfort:
Possible triggers:
My coping responses or support used:

"Things do not change; we change."
HENRY DAVID THOREAU

POWER TRANSMUTATION

I am transforming pain into power.
What challenge showed up this week?
How can I shift my perspective or response?
A lesson or strength I uncovered:

....
....
....
....
....
....
....
....
....
....
....
....
....
....
....

> *"I alone cannot change the world, but I can cast a stone across the water to create many ripples."*
>
> MOTHER TERESA

WINS, GRATITUDE & MAGIC MOMENTS

1–2 wins this week:
Who or what I'm grateful for:
A magic moment I want to remember:

FREE SPACE / DOODLE / DOWNLOAD PAGE

Use this space however you like — journal, sketch, release, or let something flow through you.

"Open your arms to change, but don't let go of your values."

DALAI LAMA

MY WEEKLY INTENTION

How am I feeling emotionally, physically & spiritually?
This week, I want to feel… (let this guide your intention)
My core focus:
Support I need this week:

"Your life does not get better by chance, it gets better by change."
JIM ROHN

BODY CHECK-IN

What is my body whispering to me?
Physical sensations I've noticed:
Energy highs/lows:
What's calling for attention or rest?

"You are not behind. You are exactly where you're meant to be."

INVISIBLE PAIN TRACKER

I'm learning to name what I feel, even when no one sees it.
Pain, tension, or emotional discomfort:
Possible triggers:
My coping responses or support used:

> "Success is something you attract by the person you become."
> JIM ROHN

POWER TRANSMUTATION

I am transforming pain into power.
What challenge showed up this week?
How can I shift my perspective or response?
A lesson or strength I uncovered:

_____
_____
_____
_____
_____
_____
_____
_____
_____
_____
_____
_____
_____
_____

> *"Small hinges swing big doors."*
>
> ROBIN SHARMA

WINS, GRATITUDE & MAGIC MOMENTS

1–2 wins this week:
Who or what I'm grateful for:
A magic moment I want to remember:

FREE SPACE / DOODLE / DOWNLOAD PAGE

Use this space however you like — journal, sketch, release, or let something flow through you.

"What you are not changing, you are choosing."
LAURIE BUCHANAN

MY WEEKLY INTENTION

How am I feeling emotionally, physically & spiritually?
This week, I want to feel... (let this guide your intention)
My core focus:
Support I need this week:

"Discipline is the bridge between goals and accomplishment."
JIM ROHN

BODY CHECK-IN

What is my body whispering to me?
Physical sensations I've noticed:
Energy highs/lows:
What's calling for attention or rest?

"Your perception creates your reality—choose wisely."

INVISIBLE PAIN TRACKER

I'm learning to name what I feel, even when no one sees it.
Pain, tension, or emotional discomfort:
Possible triggers:
My coping responses or support used:

"Your future is created by what you do today, not tomorrow."
ROBERT KIYOSAKI

POWER TRANSMUTATION

I am transforming pain into power.
What challenge showed up this week?
How can I shift my perspective or response?
A lesson or strength I uncovered:

"Don't just go through life. Grow through life."
ERIC BUTTERWORTH

WINS, GRATITUDE & MAGIC MOMENTS

1–2 wins this week:
Who or what I'm grateful for:
A magic moment I want to remember:

FREE SPACE / DOODLE / DOWNLOAD PAGE

Use this space however you like — journal, sketch, release, or let something flow through you.

"Energy flows where attention goes."

BOB PROCTOR

MY WEEKLY INTENTION

How am I feeling emotionally, physically & spiritually?
This week, I want to feel… (let this guide your intention)
My core focus:
Support I need this week:

"You can't outperform your own self-image."

MAXWELL MALTZ

BODY CHECK-IN

What is my body whispering to me?
Physical sensations I've noticed:
Energy highs/lows:
What's calling for attention or rest?

"In the middle of difficulty lies opportunity."

ALBERT EINSTEIN

INVISIBLE PAIN TRACKER

I'm learning to name what I feel, even when no one sees it.
Pain, tension, or emotional discomfort:
Possible triggers:
My coping responses or support used:

"Be so rooted in your purpose that external noise becomes irrelevant."

POWER TRANSMUTATION

I am transforming pain into power.
What challenge showed up this week?
How can I shift my perspective or response?
A lesson or strength I uncovered:

"The cave you fear to enter holds the treasure you seek."

JOSEPH CAMPBELL

WINS, GRATITUDE & MAGIC MOMENTS

1–2 wins this week:
Who or what I'm grateful for:
A magic moment I want to remember:

FREE SPACE / DOODLE / DOWNLOAD PAGE

Use this space however you like — journal, sketch, release, or let something flow through you.

CLOSING CEREMONY

Whether it took you 12 weeks or longer, the most important part is that you see yourselves, your pain, and the world around you differently.

Consider doing a mini-ritual to mark your progress i.e. write down what you used to feel about yourself, how that has now changed and safely burn the paper. That is no longer part of you, you are letting go of what no longer serves you.

Finally, how do you feel emotionally, physically, spiritually? What did you learn about yourself? What differences have you noticed? If this was impactful, consider getting another journal, I have a new one every year - we are always learning and growing and these show us how far we have come!

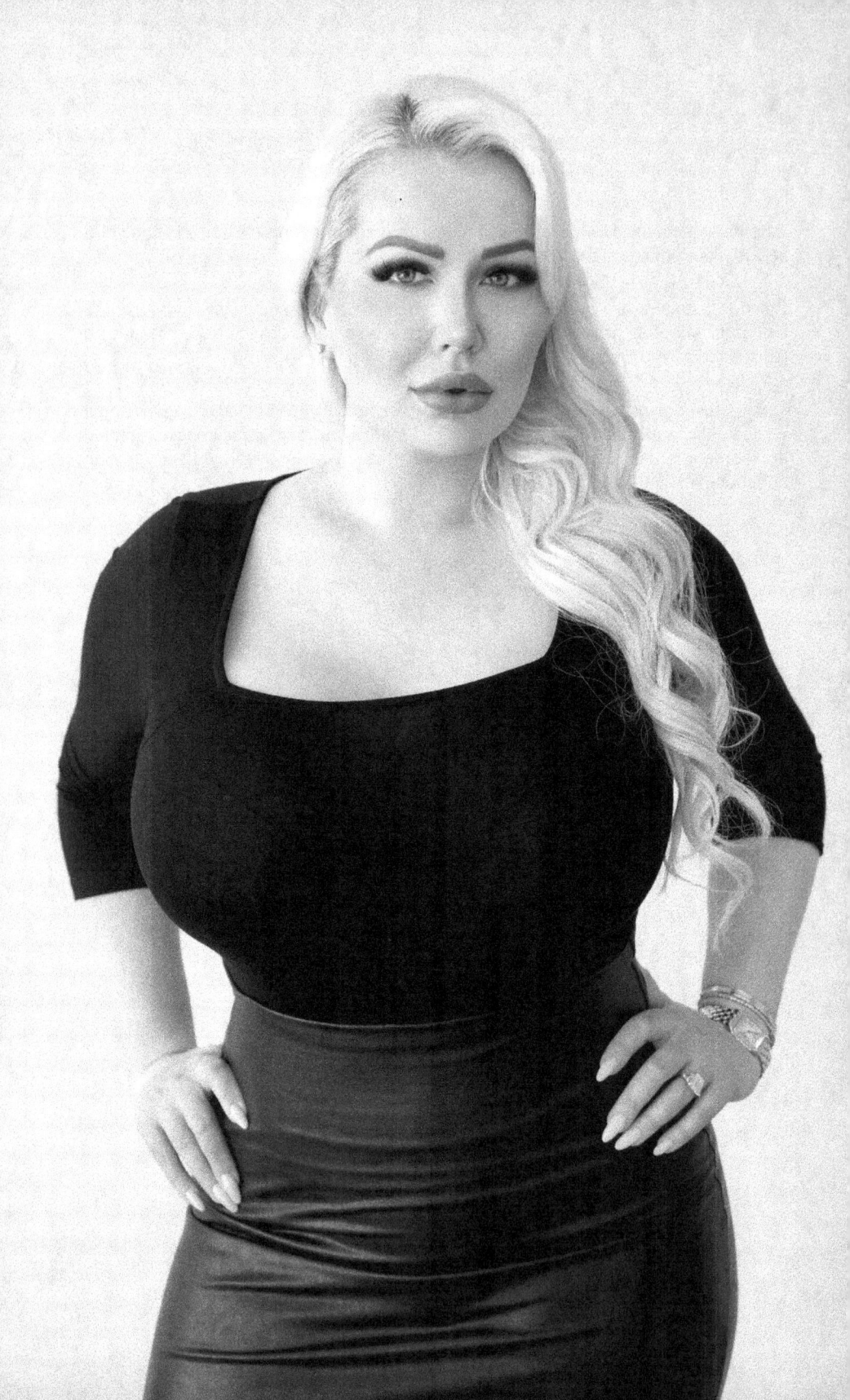

ABOUT THE AUTHOR – KATYA KARLOVA

Katya Karlova is a transformational leader, curve model, content creator, and keynote speaker whose journey from corporate executive to creative visionary has inspired thousands worldwide. Formerly an award-winning Vice President of Talent & HR for a billion-dollar health and wellness company, Katya now channels her voice into advocacy, storytelling, and powerful reinvention.

Born in the Republic of Moldova, Katya's early life ignited her passion for human rights and social justice. A proud UCLA graduate (in just three years), she went on to study at NYU, University College London, and was awarded the prestigious Erasmus Mundus Scholarship for her research on human trafficking—an issue close to her heart and homeland.

She is the founder of the Endo-Visible Foundation (www.endo-visible.com), a not-for-profit organization dedicated to raising awareness, making care affordable & accessible to all and driving global advocacy for those suffering with endometriosis and other invisible illnesses. Katya has been published on covers of fashion magazines and featured in publications like Forbes, Grazia, Men's Journal, CNBC and many others.

Her accomplishments span boardrooms and stages alike, including:

- 2019 UCLA Young Alumnus of the Year
- 2020 UCLA International Institute Commencement Speaker
- 2022 Top 50 Talent Acquisition Professionals in the U.S.
- 2024 Womenpreneur's Top 20 Most Empowering Women in the U.S.

Now a trailblazing curve model, content creator and sought after voice on healing and empowerment, Katya uses her platform to shed light on invisible illness, emotional resilience, and feminine power.

Her debut book, *Invisible Pain, Unstoppable Power*, is a deeply personal and unapologetically raw exploration of living with undiagnosed endometriosis—and rising beyond it. It is a rallying cry for every woman who has ever been dismissed, gaslit, or underestimated. Through it, Katya invites readers to reclaim their voice, their story, and their unstoppable power.

Katya continues to break barriers, champion self-expression, and speak for those still finding their words. Her mission is clear: to turn invisible pain into undeniable purpose.

NOTES

NOTES

NOTES

NOTES

NOTES

www.ingramcontent.com/pod-product-compliance
Lightning Source LLC
Chambersburg PA
CBHW060943230426
43665CB00015B/2040